Homemade Beauty: All Natural DIY Beauty Recipes Used by the World's Sexiest Celebs

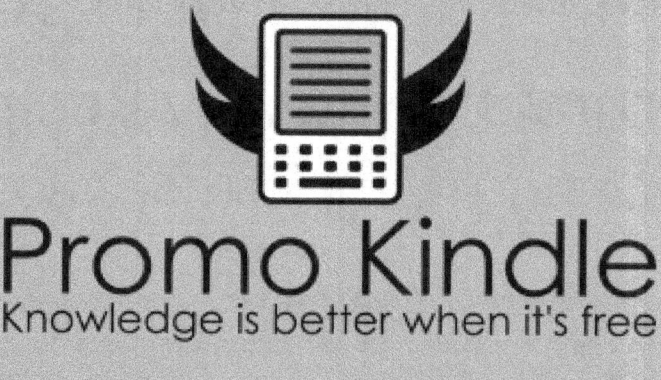

Disclaimer and Terms of Use: Effort has been made to ensure that the information in this book is accurate and complete, however, the author and the publisher do not warrant the accuracy of the information, text and graphics contained within the book due to the rapidly changing nature of science, research, known and unknown facts and internet. The Author and the publisher do not hold any responsibility for errors, omissions or contrary interpretation of the subject matter herein. This book is presented solely for motivational and informational purposes only.

Table of Contents

Rosemary mint shampoo 7

Homemade deodorant for sensitive skin 8

Sunshine Sun screen 9

Daily moisturizer 10

Face Wash 11

Honey lip moisturizer 12

Disinfectant 13

Bath salts for detox 14

Foot Rub 15

Bug rub with magnesium 16

Hand sanitizer 17

First Aid Cream 18

First Aid Spray 19

Stress sugar Rub 20

Homemade tooth paste 21

Bath salts 22

Acne cream 23

Face peel 24

Papaya Pimple cure 25

White Cream 26

Tea tree Treatment 27

Lucky lemon lacquer 28

Garlic treatment 29

Sugar treatment 30

Tea treatment 31

Rosemary mint shampoo

Ingredients:
- ½ C castile soap
- ½ C filtered water
- 14-16 drops rosemary essentials
- 2 drops peppermint drops

Directions: Add the soap to container with a flip lid, add the essential oils and water last. It's rather simple.

Homemade deodorant for sensitive skin

Ingredients:
- 6 T arrowroot powder
- 3 T shea butter
- 2 T coconut oil
- 1 T baking soda
- 2 T bentonite clay
- 10 drops essential oil

Directions: Add the butter and oil in a mixer and whisk or whip. You want to add the oil slowly and slowly add the remaining ingredients, 1/3 of the dry stuff. Then add remaining ingredients. It will look a lot like dough. Scoop the dough out and make a ground ball of dough and stuff into a glass mason jar, or likewise. You just scoop a pea size out daily and rub on arm pits.

Sunshine Sun screen

Ingredients:
- 2 oz. beeswax
- 1 oz. cocoa butter
- 1oz. shea butter
- 2 oz. coconut butter
- 2 oz. avocado oil
- 1 T zinc oxide powder
- 10 drops carrot seed essential oils
- 10 drops myrrh essential oils
- 24 drops lavender oils
- 1-2 drops sandalwood essential oil

Directions: Using double boiler combine wax, butters, and oil until melted. Remove from heat and wish with oxide you want no lumps and very smooth texture. Stir in avocado oil and other oils and whisk.

Daily moisturizer

Ingredients:
- 0-12 drop carrot seed essential oils
- 4-6 drops myrrh essential oils
- 6 drops lavender essential oils
- 4 drops frankincense oil
- ¼ C coconut oil

Directions: add everything to a mixer and whip, you want this light and fluffy. This is a great daily face moisturizer.

Face Wash

Ingredients:

- ½ tsp almond oil
- 1/3 C castile soap
- 10 drops ylang ylang essential oils
- 6 drops patchouli essential oils
- 2/3 c distilled water

Directions: Start with your soap and almond oil in a foaming soap dispenser, add oils and combine fill with water and add lid. Use this daily

Honey lip moisturizer

Ingredients:
- 2 T coconut oil
- 2 T shea butter
- ½ raw honey
- 1 T sweet almond oil
- 1 T beeswax
- 15 drops lavender essential oil
- 5 drops frankincense oil

Directions: You need empty lip balm containers (save your old ones) melt the coconut sea, honey and beeswax in a double boiler. Stir from heat and stir in almond oil. Pour melted oils into empty recycled lip balm tubes and let set.

Disinfectant

Ingredients:
- 20 drops essential oil blends
- 4 oz. spray bottle
- Distilled water
- ½ tsp salt

Directions: start with your salt in the spray bottle, then add oils let the salt absorb the oil and slowly add your water. Add lid, shake then spray.

Bath salts for detox

Ingredients:
- 3 dead salt
- 25 drops favorite essential oils
- 1 T coconut oil

Directions: Add everything in a container together and store in air tight corner. Use ½ C in bath per use.

Foot Rub

Ingredients:
- 20 drops extra virgin olive oil
- 10 drops thieves essential oil
- 10 drops oregano essential oil

Directions: add olive oil and thieves and oregano to bottle (use roll in bottle) apple as needed to your feet

Bug rub with magnesium

Ingredients:
- ½ C shea butter
- ½ C coconut oil
- 1/3 C magnesium oil
- 50 drops peace essential oils

Directions: start with warming the coconut oil and shea butter in a glass bowl. Let simmer, once melted allow to cool, and it will start setting. You can scoop or spoon it into hand mixer and whip. You want a nice "cool whip" setting for your rub. Store in air tight jar.

Hand sanitizer

Ingredients:
- 2 T aloe Vera
- 2 T water
- 1/8 tsp vitamin E oil
- 5 drops thieves oil

Directions: Combine everything thing and rub on hands.

First Aid Cream

Ingredients:
- 4 T rose ointment
- 5 drops lavender
- 3 drops melaluea alternifolia
- 2 drops dorado azul

Directions: start with small saucepan with 1" water and let simmer add 4 T of rose and add to jar. You want to let these slowly melt to a liquid state. Let sit for about one hour.

First Aid Spray

Ingredients:
- 3 drops lavender
- 2 drops melalueca
- 1 drop dorado azul
- ¼ tsp. salt
- 4 oz. distilled water

Directions: Add salt to spray bottle, drop oils and allow salt to absorb. Fill bottle with water and shake well.

Stress sugar Rub

Ingredients:
- 1 C sugar
- ¼ C olive oil
- 2 T raw honey
- 40 drops essential oil for stress

Directions: Combine everything in glass jar and melt away. This really works

Homemade tooth paste

Ingredients:
- ¾ C filtered water
- ¼ C apple cider vinegar
- 40 drops peppermint essential oil

Directions: Mix water and vinegar in spray bottle, add oils and mist on your face in the morning or at night or both.

Bath salts

Ingredients:
- 3 C dead sea salts
- 25 drops essential oils
- T coconut oil

Directions: Combine everything and store in air tight container

Acne cream

Ingredients:
- 2 T honey
- 1 tsp cinnamon
- Paper towels

Directions: Rinse face with water and dry, mix the two ingredients and leave on your face for about 101-2 minutes. Rinse and dry your face.

Face peel

Ingredients:
- 2 orange peels
- Water

Directions: rinse and dry your face, grind orange peels, in a blender if you have one. Add water to get a paste consistency. Add to your entire face or problem areas and let sit for 20 minutes or so, and scrap or wipe cream off and pat dry.

Papaya Pimple cure

Ingredients:
- 1 papaya (Fresh is best)

Directions: rinse your face and dry, mash up papaya and apply to your face. Leave on for face for about 20-24 minutes and remove. Pat ry.

White Cream

Ingredients:
- 3 egg whites
- Bowl

Directions: Make sure face is clean and dry. Try starting with 2 or 3 egg whites and whisk. Let egg whites get frothy add extra attention to troubled areas, and let sit for 20 minutes and then use warm water and rag to remove mask.

Tea tree Treatment

Ingredients:
- Tea tree oil
- Water

Directions:

Make sure your face is clean and dry. Add one drop oil per 9 parts water. Use a Q-tip for best results. You just want to apply this to trouble areas. If that isn't enough you can cut back on diluting the tree oil. Let sit for 1-15 minutes and wipe clean.

Lucky lemon lacquer

Ingredients:
- 1 T lemon juice (fresh is best)
- Yogurt

Directions: make sure face is clean and dry, use Q-tips to your fingers to apply to your face in trouble acne areas. Let sit and wipe clean. You can use the yogurt to dilute the lemon juice. It will help alleviate any burning you may feel.

Garlic treatment

Ingredients:
- 2 garlic cloves
- Aloe Vera gel

Directions: extract garlic juice and mix with1 tsp water and let cloves sit in water for a few minutes, using fingertip, cotton ball or Q tip apply to your troubled areas and let sit for a few minutes and wipe clean.

Sugar treatment

Ingredients:
- 1 ½ C sugar
- 1 ½ C brown sugar
- 3 T sea salt
- ½ C olive oil (extra virgin olive oil)
- 10 T vanilla extract
- 1 vanilla bean

Directions: Mix the brown sugar and white sugar together sea salts a little at a time and scarped vanilla beans. Add 2 C of this mixture and pack well. Add oil and let it sit and marinade more or less. Ix rest of ingredients and let sit. Apply to face and let sit for 10-14 minutes and rinse.

Tea treatment

Ingredients:
- ½ C water
- 1 green teabag

Directions: Make sure your face is clean and dry. Add tea to bowl of boiling water. Let sit for around 5 minutes and strain. You can add this to a spray bottle and use as needed. Let it sit on your face for around 3 minutes before rinsing, or you can leave it on your face.